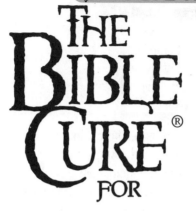

THE BIBLE CURE® FOR

DIABETES

DON COLBERT, M.D.

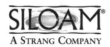

SILOAM®
A Strang Company

THE BIBLE CURE FOR DIABETES
by Don Colbert, M.D.
Published by Siloam
A Strang Company
600 Rinehart Road
Lake Mary, Florida 32746
www.siloam.com

Library of Congress Catalog Card Number:
99-93490

International Standard Book Number:
0-88419-648-8

This book is not intended to provide medical advice or to take the place of medical advice and treatment from your personal physician. Readers are advised to consult their own doctors or other qualified health professionals regarding the treatment of their medical problems. Neither the publisher nor the author takes any responsibility for any possible consequences from any treatment, action or application of medicine, supplement, herb or preparation to any person reading or following the information in this book. If readers are taking prescription medications, they should consult with their physicians and not take themselves off of medicines to start supplementation without the proper supervision of a physician.

04 05 06 07— 18 17 16 15
Printed in the United States of America

There's Hope
for Diabetes

God's desire for you is to feel better and live longer and He will help you reach that goal! By picking up this Bible Cure booklet, you have taken an exciting first step toward renewed energy, health and vigor.

You may be confronting the greatest physical challenge of your life. But with faith in God and good nutrition, combined with cutting-edge alternative natural remedies, I believe it will be your greatest victory! God revealed His divine will for each of us through the apostle John who wrote, "Dear friend, I am praying that all is well with you and that *your body is as healthy as I know your soul is*" (3 John 2, emphasis added).

Nearly two thousand years later, more than

15.7 million Americans suffer from a disease called diabetes—and a third of them don't even know it! This disease ranks as the seventh leading cause of death in America.[1]

Surely we are missing God's best for us. But how? A closer look will reveal some hopeful answers. You see, your body is "fearfully and wonderfully made," and it contains a specialized gland called the pancreas. This gland secretes digestive enzymes and vital hormones that regulate the amount of sugar in the bloodstream.

The most well-known of these hormones is insulin. The body converts the food we eat into a form of sugar known as glucose and distributes it to the cells of the body through the bloodstream. Each cell is a self-contained structure with a delicate environment, so the cell walls will not allow outside substances to enter without a "key" or "gatekeeper" to make an opening. Insulin is the body's key that allows glucose to leave the bloodstream and enter a cell.

Under normal circumstances, the pancreas efficiently manages the level of sugar in our blood day after day and year after year without incident. Frankly, most people rarely think about their pancreas unless a problem develops. When the pancreas produces too little insulin, one form of diabetes may result. You probably know someone with diabetes who takes insulin shots every day—perhaps you are one of these diabetics. These individuals have to carefully watch what they eat so they can avoid going into diabetic seizures or worse. Good medical treatment, good nutrition and other healthy lifestyle choices can significantly benefit the first type of diabetes.

Few people realize that two different types of diabetes exist. A second type of this disease, which we will discuss in detail later, can be completely prevented or successfully managed with a healthy diet and wise lifestyle choices. Regardless of which type of diabetes you or a loved one may have, God can totally heal either one without effort or difficulty. I've known many people who have been completely healed of diabetes by the miracle-working power of God. I have also witnessed many others whose lives have been dramatically improved through healthy lifestyle choices and natural treatments.

So, as you begin to read through the pages of this booklet, get ready to feel better! This Bible Cure booklet is filled with hope and encouragement for understanding how to keep your body fit and healthy. In this book, you will

uncover God's divine plan of health
for body, soul and spirit
through modern medicine, good nutrition
and the medicinal power
of Scripture and prayer.

You will find key Scripture passages throughout this book that will help you focus on the healing power of God.

These divine promises will empower your prayers and redirect your thoughts to line up with God's plan of divine health for you—a plan that includes victory over diabetes or its prevention altogether. In this Bible Cure book, you will learn how to overcome diabetes in the following chapters:

There is much we can do to prevent or defeat diabetes. Now it is time to run to the battle with fresh confidence, renewed determination and the wonderful knowledge that God is real, He is alive and His power is greater than any sickness or disease.

It is my prayer that these practical suggestions for health, nutrition and fitness will bring wholeness to your life. May they deepen your fellowship with God and strengthen your ability to worship and serve Him.

—Don Colbert, M.D.

A Bible Cure Prayer FOR YOU

Dear heavenly Father, You have declared in Your Word that I am healed by the stripes Your Son, Jesus Christ, bore on His back. For Your Word says that "He was pierced through for our transgressions. He was crushed for our iniquities. The chastening of our well-being fell upon Him. And by His scourging we are healed" (Isa. 53:5, NAS).

Father, Your Son Jesus has given us the authority to use His name when we pray.

This is the same name by which You spoke into being the heavens and the earth long ago. In that precious name I declare that Your Word is true: I am healed by the stripes Jesus bore on His back. Whether I must wait for a minute, a week, a year or a lifetime for my physical healing to be complete, by faith I will praise You for it as if it were already complete. I thank You for a healthy pancreas that produces and properly regulates the insulin levels in my body. Help me make wise choices and follow the guidelines in Your Word concerning food choices, lifestyle, prayer and a thought life that is saturated with Your living Word. Thank You for hearing and answering my prayer so I will be free to serve You with my whole mind, body, soul and strength. Amen.

Chapter 1

Know Your Enemy

I have good news for you: Not only did God heal the sick in the days of the Bible. He still heals today! He has also given us a wealth of proven Bible principles and invaluable medical knowledge about the human body. You can control the symptoms and potentially damaging effects of diabetes while you seek Him for total healing. You are destined to be more than a victim. You are destined to be a victor in this battle!

Your first order of battle is to *know your enemy.* Measure its strengths and plan for its defeat. The enemy called diabetes comes in two forms.

Type 1 Diabetes

Type 1 diabetes is insulin-dependent diabetes. In

this type the pancreas cannot make insulin. Approximately 10 to 20 percent of all diabetics have Type 1 diabetes and require insulin for their entire lives.[1] This form of the disease usually strikes during the childhood years.

Individuals battling with the insulin-dependent form of diabetes will greatly benefit from the nutritional information and biblical truths shared in this book. Continue to follow all of the advice of your physician, and consult him or her before making any lifestyle and nutritional changes. In addition, determine to believe God—who created your pancreas in the first place—for a miraculous touch of healing power. The Word of God says, "For nothing will be impossible with God" (Luke 1:37, NAS).

> *Don't you realize that all of you together are the temple of God and that the Spirit of God lives in you? God will bring ruin upon anyone who ruins this temple. For God's temple is holy, and you Christians are that temple.*
> —1 CORINTHIANS 3:16–17

Remember that faith is not a feeling or an emotion; faith is a choice. Specifically ask the Lord to heal your pancreas and restore its ability to manufacture insulin, or if necessary, ask Him to create what was never there in the first place. Don't let discouragement set in—it is as easy for the Creator to make a new pancreas as it is to repair a damaged one!

Type 2 Diabetes

Type 2 diabetes is non-insulin-dependent diabetes. In Type 2 diabetes the pancreas does make insulin, but the body cannot use the insulin properly. This form of the disease is sometimes called adult-onset diabetes because its victims tend to contract the disease in their adult years. However, our nation's taste for a high-sugar, high-fat diet seems to have removed the age barrier. The medical community now reports that this form of diabetes accounts for a growing number of juvenile cases.

With this form of diabetes, the insulin levels in the blood are usually elevated (which means the pancreas is producing more insulin than normal). At the same time, the cells are resistant to the insulin because the insulin receptors on the surfaces of these cells do not function properly. They no longer recognize or accept insulin as a key, so more insulin is needed to "force the issue" so sugar can move from the blood to the starving cells. That means that an excessive amount of insulin is needed to keep the blood sugar in the normal range. When the system breaks down, blood sugar levels get dangerously high (this is called hyperglycemia) while the body's cells are starving for lack of the blood sugar that is surrounding them.

Approximately 80 to 90 percent of diabetics are Type 2 diabetics, and insulin resistance is one of the greatest enemies to their health if God does not heal them outright. This is usually a very manageable problem, but it is complicated by the fact that obesity is one of the most important factors leading to insulin resistance. That means that obese people with Type 2 diabetes must fight a battle on two fronts: they must drop their weight down to safer levels while they also carefully monitor and control their blood sugar levels. This also means that Type 2 diabetics require:

- a diet that is low in starch
- a diet that has no sugar

Symptoms You Must Not Ignore

As with most diseases, early detection of diabetes is very important. Silent enemies sometimes inflict the most damage. Fortunately, Type 2 diabetes has some telltale symptoms that may tip you off to a problem that needs attention:

- urinary frequency
- extreme thirst
- feelings of edginess, fatigue and often feeling sick to your stomach
- being overweight (defined as 20 to 30 percent higher than the ideal weight for your body frame, height and age)
- increased appetite
- repeated or hard-to-heal infections of the skin, gums, vagina or bladder
- blurred vision
- tingling or loss of feeling in the hands or feet
- dry, itchy skin

Some of these symptoms may occur from time to time simply because you drink too much liquid one night, eat some spicy food or stay up too late. However, if you experience one or more of these symptoms on a regular basis, make an appointment with your physician and get the facts about the symptoms. Then you can apply the truths of

God's Word to the situation. Above all, don't give in to fear or apathy. Never mistake ignorance or fear for true spirituality.

Treatable and Beatable

As with most diseases, serious health complications occur when someone with diabetes fails to do anything about this treatable and beatable disease. The more serious complications of diabetes include diabetic retinopathy (a retina

> *And God said, "Look! I have given you the seed-bearing plants throughout the earth and all the fruit trees for your food. And I have given all the grasses and other green plants to the animals and birds for their food." And so it was.*
> —GENESIS 1:29–30

disorder that is the leading cause of blindness in the U.S.), cataracts, diabetic neuropathy (a degeneration of the peripheral nervous system that leads to tingling, numbness, pain and weakness usually in extremities such as the legs and feet), kidney disease and arteriosclerosis, which is a narrowing of the arteries due to fatty deposits on the artery walls.

Since diabetes severely affects the body's circulatory system, it may harm or overload many of the major organs and systems that interact with or depend on the circulatory system for energy (food), elimination of wastes and oxygen. Diabetics—particularly those who fail to control their insulin and blood sugar levels through proper diet, exercise and lifestyle choices—are much more prone to heart disease, heart attacks, kidney disease (one of the main causes of death in diabetics), diabetic foot ulcers (usually due to a poor blood supply) and peripheral nerve disease of the feet.

Avoid These Health Complications

The National Institutes of Health says that diabetes contributes to the following diseases and health complications:[2]

- *Heart disease.* This is the leading cause of diabetes-related deaths. Adults with diabetes have heart disease death rates that are about two to four times higher than those of adults without diabetes because the disease accelerates blood vessel deterioration and can greatly impair proper blood flow to the oxygen-dependent muscles of the heart.

- *Stroke.* The risk of a stroke is two to four times higher in people with diabetes because the disease impairs the circulatory system overall while increasing the risk of blood clots to sensitive areas such as the brain.

- *High blood pressure.* An estimated 60 to 65 percent of people with diabetes have high blood pressure. The cause should be obvious, considering the effects of diabetes on the cardiovascular and circulatory system mentioned earlier.

- *Blindness.* Diabetes is the leading cause of new cases of blindness in adults between twenty and seventy-four years old. Diabetic retinopathy causes from 12,000 to 24,000 new cases of blindness each year. These conditions stem from the increased "blood plaque" activity fostered by diabetes, when particles of plaque comprised of fat and other deposits invade and block the tiny arteries and capillaries of the eye. The flow of blood is unable to get to the cells, and they eventually die, causing blindness.

- *Kidney disease.* Diabetes is the leading

cause of end-stage kidney disease, accounting for about 40 percent of new cases. In 1995, 27,851 people with diabetes developed advanced kidney disease. In that same year, a total of 98,872 people with diabetes underwent dialysis or had kidney transplants.

- *Nervous system damage.* About 60 to 70 percent of people with diabetes have mild to severe forms of nervous system damage (called diabetic neuropathy), which often includes impaired sensation or pain in the feet or hands, slowed digestion of food in the stomach, carpal tunnel syndrome and other nerve problems.

- *Amputations.* Severe forms of diabetic nerve disease are a major contributing cause of lower extremity amputations. More than half of lower limb amputations in the United States occur among people with diabetes. From 1993 to 1995, about 67,000 amputations were performed each year among people with diabetes. The lower extremities are more susceptible to the circulatory impairment caused by diabetes simply because they are further from the heart. The nutrients and oxygen in the bloodstream must make their way through a much greater distance of blood vessels and capillaries to nourish cells in the feet and toes.

- *Dental disease.* Dental disease, in the form of periodontal disease (a type of gum disease that can lead to tooth loss), occurs with greater frequency and severity among people with diabetes. Periodontal disease has been reported to occur among 30 percent of people nineteen years of age or older with Type 1, insulin-dependent diabetes.

- *Pregnancy complications.* The rate of major congenital malformations in babies born to women with preexisting diabetes varies from zero to five percent among women who receive preconception care. The rate rises to 10 percent among women who do not receive preconception care. Between 3 and 5 percent of pregnancies among women with diabetes result in the death of the newborn; this rate for pregnancies of women who do not have diabetes is 1.5 percent.

- *Flu and pneumonia.* Diabetics are also more susceptible to flu and pneumonia.

The Good News

After reading through all of these dismal complications, you may feel like tiny David when he stood before the nine-foot giant called Goliath. Don't give in to fear. These are the complications that most often affect Type 1 diabetic sufferers whose blood sugar levels are not controlled through proper diet and exercise.

In the face of these medical facts, your goal is to take advantage of the wealth of wisdom in God's Word and in the medical knowledge He has given us over the centuries to avoid these complications altogether by making wise choices. Most importantly, your primary goal is to take hold of the healing Jesus bought for you when He suffered under the Roman lash.

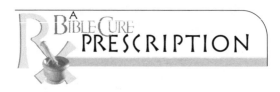

Faith Builder

He was pierced through for our transgressions, He was crushed for our iniquities; the chastening of our well-being fell upon Him, and by His scourging we are healed.

—ISAIAH 53:5, NAS

Write out this verse and insert your own name into it: "He was pierced through for _____'s transgressions, He was crushed for _____'s iniquities; the chastening of _____'s well-being fell on Him, and by His scourgings _____ is healed!"

Write out a personal prayer to Jesus Christ thanking Him for exchanging His health for your pain. Thank Him for taking the power of sickness onto His own body so that He could purchase your healing from diabetes.

_____

_____

_____

_____

Chapter 2

Battle Diabetes
With Good Nutrition

The same God who skillfully designed your body as an incredible, living machine and created your pancreas to produce insulin also designed the human body to operate at peak efficiency and health when it is supplied with proper nutrition. If you are a diabetic, what you eat makes all the difference in the world!

Ask God to give you a new way of looking at nutrition. You'll be surprised at the way your thinking about food begins to change. First, and most importantly, you must avoid eating foods with a *high glycemic index.*

What Is the Glycemic Index?

The glycemic index measures how quickly

various carbohydrates enter the bloodstream. If the glycemic index for a certain food is high, then it will raise your blood sugar levels much faster (this is bad). High blood sugar levels, in turn, increase the amount of insulin that will be secreted by Type 2 diabetics to bring the blood sugar level back into balance.

White bread has a glycemic index of 95. Generally speaking, the more a food is processed, the greater will be its glycemic index. This is because processed food is usually broken down faster during digestion. For example, French bread has a very high glycemic index because it is processed more than other breads. Refried beans have a higher glycemic index than regular black beans or kidney beans.

> *Don't worry about anything; instead, pray about everything. Tell God what you need, and thank him for all he has done. If you do this, you will experience God's peace, which is far more wonderful than the human mind can understand. His peace will guard your hearts and minds as you live in Christ Jesus.*
> —PHILIPPIANS 4:6–7

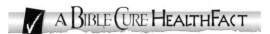

Glycemic Index of Foods

EXTREMELY HIGH
(GREATER THAN 100)

GRAIN-BASED FOODS

Puffed rice
Millet
French bread

Corn flakes
Instant rice

VEGETABLES

Cooked parsnips
Instant potatoes
Borad beans (Fava Beans)

Baked russet potato
Cooked carrots

SIMPLE SUGARS

Maltose
Honey

GLYCEMIC STANDARD=100

White bread

HIGH (80–100)

GRAIN-BASED FOODS

Wheat bread
Whole-meal bread
Shredded wheat
Rye bread, crispbread
Brown rice
Sweet corn

Grape Nuts
Corn tortilla
Muesli
Rye bread, whole
Porridge oats
White rice

VEGETABLES

Mashed potatoes	Broiled new potato

FRUITS

Apricots	Raisins
Banana	Papaya
Mango	

SNACKS

Corn chips	Mars bar
Crackers	Cookies
Pastry	Low-fat ice cream

MODERATELY HIGH (60–80)

GRAIN-BASED FOODS

Buckwheat	All Bran
Pumpernickel bread	Bulgur
White macaroni	White spaghetti
Brown spaghetti	

VEGETABLES

Yam	Sweet potato
Green peas, marrowfat	Frozen green peas
Canned baked beans	Canned kidney beans

FRUITS

Fruit cocktail	Grapefruit juice
Orange juice	Pineapple juice
Canned pears	Grapes

SNACKS

Oatmeal cookies	Potato chips
Sponge cake	

MODERATE (40–60)

Vegetables

Haricot (white) beans	Tomato soup
Brown beans	Lima beans
Dried green peas	Chickpeas (garbanzo)
Butter beans	Black-eyed peas
Kidney beans	Black beans

Fruits

Orange	Apple juice
Pears	Apple

Dairy

Yogurt	High-fat ice cream
Whole milk	2 percent milk
Skim milk	

LOW (LESS THAN 40)

Grain-based food

Barley

Vegetables

Red lentils	Canned soybeans

Fruits

Peaches	Plums

Simple sugars

Fructose

Snacks

Peanuts

Foods with a high glycemic index (which means 70 or over) are capable of raising the blood sugar quickly and therefore insulin levels. Foods with high glycemic index levels that you need to avoid include instant potatoes, instant rice, French bread, white bread, corn, oats, white rice, rye bread, cereals (such as Corn Flakes or Puffed Rice), baked potatoes, mashed potatoes, cooked carrots, glucose (sugar found naturally in foods like fruit), honey, sucrose (sugar naturally extracted from cane and beets), raisins, dried fruit, candy bars, crackers, cookies, ice cream and pastries. If you are diabetic, you should either eat these foods very rarely or avoid them completely.

Puffed rice cakes have one of the highest glycemic indexes, yet people on diets commonly eat them. Remember that high-glycemic foods and high-density carbohydrates raise blood sugar quickly, which raises insulin levels. When this occurs over time, the flood of insulin released causes the blood cells to become resistant to receiving it. You might say that these high-glycemic foods are more harmful than poison to an individual at risk for Type 2 diabetes.

In the early stages of Type 2 diabetes, the pancreas is always producing too much insulin. As the disease progresses, the pancreas's insulin-producing cells eventually wear out from overwork! Individuals with a family history of diabetes are much more prone to developing Type 2 diabetes. Genetic patterns as well as eating habits are passed down through families. After years of eating high-glycemic foods, the high insulin levels in the bodies of these individuals finally catch up with them. If this describes your family, your key to keeping your health is avoiding high-glycemic foods.

If you already are a Type 2 diabetic, your pancreas may be producing about four times as much insulin as a non-diabetic's pancreas. The key to correcting the blood cells' resistance to insulin is following the proper diet. You must decrease or avoid high-

> *If you will listen carefully to the voice of the LORD your God and do what is right in his sight, obeying his commands and laws, then I will not make you suffer the diseases I sent on the Egyptians; for I am the LORD who heals you.*
> —EXODUS 15:26

density, high-glycemic starches, such as breads, white rice, potatoes and corn, and decrease fats, including saturated fats, and fried foods. If you will do this, your cells will actually recover. They will begin to regain their sensitivity to insulin. You hold the key.

The Bible and Fats

> *You must serve only the LORD your God. If you do, I will bless you with food and water, and I will keep you healthy.*
> —EXODUS 23:25

Interestingly, eating fats is condemned in the Bible. God commands: "You must never eat any fat or blood. This is a permanent law for you and all your desendants, wherever they may live" (Lev. 3:17). God created our bodies and knows how they have been designed to function best. I encourage you to substitute extra-virgin olive oil and canola oil for butter, cream and other fats. Always choose low-fat portions of meat as well.

Fantastic Fiber

Another important way you can battle diabetes through nutrition is to increase the fiber in your diet. Dietary fiber is extremely important in helping to control diabetes. Fiber slows down digestion and the absorption of carbohydrates. This allows for a more gradual rise in blood sugar.

If you have diabetes, most of the carbohydrate calories you eat should come from fruits and vegetables. Fruits and vegetables contain large amounts of fiber. The more soluble fiber in your diet, the better blood sugar control your body will have.

Water-soluble fibers are found in oat bran, seeds such as psyllium (the primary ingredient in Metamucil), fruits and vegetables (especially apples and pears), beans and nuts. You should try to take in at least 30–35 grams of fiber a day. You also should take the fiber with meals in order to prevent rapid rises in blood sugar.

> *So I tell you, don't worry about everyday life whether you have enough food, drink, and clothes. Doesn't life consist of more than food and clothing? Look at the birds. They don't need to plant or harvest or put food in barns because your heavenly Father feeds them. And you are far more valuable to him than they are.*
> —MATTHEW 6:25–26

Increasing Fiber in Your Diet

You might try the following ideas to increase the fiber in your diet:

- Eat at least five servings of fruits and vegetables each day. Fruits and vegetables that are high in fiber include:

Apples	Peas	Broccoli
Spinach	Berries	Pears
Brussels sprouts	Beans (all types)	Parsnips
Prunes	Carrots	Lentils

- Replace white bread with whole-grain breads and cereals. Eat brown rice instead of white rice. Examples of these foods include:

Bran muffins	Oatmeal	Brown rice

Multiple-grain cereals, cooked or dry
100% whole-wheat or whole-grain bread

- Eat dry bran cereal for breakfast. Check labels on the packages for the amounts of dietary fiber in each brand. Some cereals may have less fiber than you think.

- Add $\frac{1}{4}$ cup of wheat bran (miller's bran) to foods such as cooked cereal or applesauce.

- Eat cooked beans a few times a week.

Many foods contain dietary fiber (the part of food that resists digestion by the body). Eating foods that are high in fiber can not only help relieve some problems with diabetes but also may help lower your cholesterol and even prevent heart disease and certain types of cancer.

A Word of Caution

Make small changes in your diet over a period of time to help prevent bloating, cramping or gas. Start by adding one of the items listed above to your diet, then wait several days or even a week before making another change. If one change doesn't seem to work for you, try a different one.

It's important to drink more fluids when you increase the amount of fiber you eat. Drink at least two additional glasses of water a day when you increase your fiber intake.

This information provides a general overview on dietary fiber and may not apply to everyone. Talk to your family doctor to find out if this information applies to you and to get more information on this subject. I have included some menu planning tips in chapter four to help you increase your fiber intake as you plan your menus.

What About Bread?

Americans love white bread, coffee and hot dogs. However, processing white bread removes all the bran and germ, along with

> *You must never eat any fat or blood. This is a permanent law for you and all your descendants, wherever they may live.*
> —LEVITICUS 3:17

approximately 80 percent of the nutrients and virtually all the fiber. Bleaching the flour destroys even more vitamins. Sugar and hydrogenated fats are added, right along with manufactured vitamins. In the end you get a product that is pure starch— stripped of the fiber and nutritional value of whole grain breads. Add water to white bread, and it forms a sticky, glue-like substance. Is there any wonder why this food takes double the amount of time to be eliminated from the body?

America's romance with processed foods, such as breads, potatoes and other grains, is one of the main reasons we see diabetes increasing every year at alarming rates.

Today the best choices of bread are the sprouted breads found in most health food stores. I personally choose Ezekiel bread, which is made of the sprouts of wheat, barley and other grains.

Remember, even if breads at the supermarket are called whole-grain breads, they also contain sugar and hydrogenated fats and are processed in such a way that they still have fairly high glycemic indexes. Therefore, if my diabetic patients request bread, I recommend that they have only a small amount of sprouted bread, such as Ezekiel bread, in the morning or at lunch. Following is a recipe for Ezekiel bread. Try it. You'll love the taste!

> *I know how to live on almost nothing or with everything. I have learned the secret of living in every situation, whether it is with a full stomach or empty, with plenty or little. For I can do everything with the help of Christ who gives me the strength I need.*
> —PHILIPPIANS 4:12–13

A BIBLE CURE RECIPE

EZEKIEL BREAD

2½ cups whole wheat
1½ cups whole rye
½ cup barley
¼ cup millet
¼ cup lentils
2 tablespoons great northern beans (uncooked)
2 tablespoons red kidney beans (uncooked)
2 tablespoons pinto beans (uncooked)

Measure and combine all the above ingredients into a large bowl. This makes 8 cups of flour. Use 4 cups per batch of bread. Pour these ingredients into a flour mill and grind. The flour should be the consistency of regular flour. Coarse flour may cause digestion problems. Measure 4 cups of flour. Store remaining 4 cups in freezer for future use.

Measure 1 cup lukewarm water (110–115 degrees) in a small mixing bowl. Add to the water, stirring to dissolve, 1 teaspoon honey and 2 tablespoons Red Star yeast or 2 tablespoons of any other brand (2 packages). Set aside and let yeast grow five to ten minutes.

In a large mixing bowl, combine the following:

Flour
¼ cup extra-virgin olive oil
½ cup honey
1 cup warm water

Add yeast to above mixture. Stir until well mixed. Mixture should have the consistency of slightly heavy cornbread. Spread out evenly in a 11" x 15" x 1" pan sprayed with olive oil. Let mixture rise in a warm place for 1 hour. Bake at 375 degrees for approximately 30 minutes. Check for doneness. Bread should not be doughy; it should have the consistency somewhat like baked cornbread.

If you do not have a flour mill, you can order Ezekiel flour from a baking catalog, such as the Baker's Catalogue (1-800-827-6836). If such flours are used, however, the texture of the bread will be entirely different from the above recipe.

A Final Word

In summary, proper diet is still the cornerstone for treating diabetes. If you are a Type 1 diabetic you must avoid sugar altogether and dramatically limit starches. Limit fruit as well, because it can also raise the blood sugar dramatically. High-fiber foods such as legumes (beans) and root vegetables (uncooked carrots) will help lower blood sugar. Type 1 diabetics must also avoid fruit juices. Their diet should be closely monitored by their physician or dietician.

However, Type 2 diabetics can benefit from fruits that are high in fiber, such as apples and pears, if they are used conservatively.

The most important dietary advice is to avoid sugar and to dramatically limit high-density starches, including breads, pasta, potatoes, corn, white rice and other highly processed foods.

Getting God's Help

Your Creator, the God of infinite power and limitless creative imagination, is also the One who will help you throughout your life if you let Him. His creative genius surrounds you every day. He doesn't expect you to be perfect, just to receive Him into your life. Have you ever felt that you've blown it in the way you eat and the way you live? God is ready to forgive and help you do better. His power to forgive is as great as His power to love. Never forget how much He loves you.

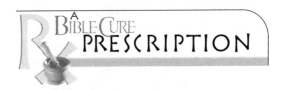

Toward a New Nutritional Lifestyle

List the top five problem foods on your own glycemic index:

_____

_____

_____

_____

_____

List five healthy food choices you will make this week instead:

_____

_____

_____

_____

_____

In what ways do you need God's help to change your eating habits?

_____

_____

_____

_____

_____

Write out a Bible cure prayer asking for God's help in making these changes.

_____

_____

_____

_____

_____

_____

_____

_____

_____

_____

Chapter 3

Battle Diabetes
With Exercise

Your body, the dwelling place of God's Spirit, needs to be protected and kept healthy. You must take courage and continually battle diabetes, because it can weaken and damage other organs in your body.

I cannot stress enough how important it is to overcome your diabetes with exercise. Exercise holds special benefits for diabetics. By helping muscles to take up glucose from the bloodstream and use it for energy, exercise prevents sugar from accumulating in the blood. By burning calories, exercise helps control weight, an important factor in the management of Type 2 diabetes.

Exercise is extremely important for both Type 1

and Type 2 diabetics. All diabetics should consult with their physicians before beginning an exercise program. Begin with walking briskly three to four times a week for at least twenty minutes. Then walk at a pace that is comfortable for you. However, you should walk briskly enough so that you cannot sing, but not so briskly that you cannot talk.

Here's a walking program to help get you started. Don't look at walking as work. Instead, see it as a special time to be alone with God, surrounded by the wonders of His creation.

> *When you sit down to dine with a ruler, consider carefully what is before you; and put a knife to your throat, if you are a man of great appetite. Do not desire his delicacies, for it is deceptive food.*
> —PROVERBS 23:1–3, NAS

A Simple Walking Program

(NOTE: Each column indicates the number of minutes to walk. Complete three exercise sessions each week. If you find a particular week's pattern tiring, repeat it before going on to the next pattern. You do not have to complete the walking program in twelve weeks.)

Week	—Walk	—Walk Briskly	—Walk	—Minutes
1	5	5	5	15
2	5	7	5	17
3	5	9	5	19
4	5	11	5	21
5	5	13	5	23
6	5	15	5	25
7	5	18	5	28
8	5	20	5	30
9	5	23	5	33
10	5	26	5	36
11	5	28	5	38
12	5	30	5	40

Week 13 and thereafter: Check your pulse periodically to see if you are exercising within your target zone. As you get more in shape, try exercising within the upper range of your target zone. Gradually increase your brisk walking time to 30 to 60 minutes, three or four times a week. Remember that your goal is to get the benefits you are seeking and enjoy your activity.

You can also obtain a heart rate monitor that straps around your chest to calculate your heart rate.

Your Predicted Heart Rate

Calculate your predicted heart rate using this formula:

220 minus [your age] = _____

x .65 = _____ x .80 = _____

Calculate your target heart zone using this formula:

220 minus [your age] = _____

x .65 = _____

[This is your minimum.]

220 minus [your age] = _____

x .80 = _____

[This is your maximum.]

This example may help: To calculate the target heart zone for a 40-year-old man, subtract the age (40) from 220 (220- 40=180). Multiply 180 by .65, which equals 117. Then multiply 180 by .80, which equals 144. A 40-year-old man's target heart rate zone is 117–144 beats per minute.

Once you have determined your desired heart rate range, write down your actual heart rate after each walking session or other exercise.

Sticking With It

Many people find that difficult as it is to start an exercise program, it is even more difficult to stick with it. Here's a tip: Make your walking program a vital part of your day. Too many people get into trouble when they save exercising for their spare time. If you wait until you can get around to it, you probably never will.

Choose an exercise activity that you truly enjoy. Walking is only one suggestion. Have you tried ballroom dancing? Or backpacking? Perhaps you've always pictured yourself on a tennis court? Surely there is an activity that you always thought you'd like to try. Now's the time— try it. If you enjoy it, then stick with it.

> *Have you found honey? Eat only what you need, lest you have it in excess . . . It is not good to eat much honey.*
> —PROVERBS 25:16, 27, NAS

In addition, most people feel calm and have a sense of well-being after they exercise. You can actually walk off your anxieties. People who exercise feel better about themselves, look better, feel more energetic and are more productive at work.

Now, Take the Offensive!

Take the offensive and follow the positive steps suggested in this chapter. You will discover how effective God's wisdom can be in both the spiritual and natural realms. God heals in many ways, whether through supernatural means or through the more gradual—but equally divine—means of proper nutrition, exercise and biblical life choices.

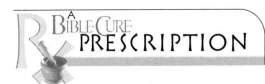

**Battling Diabetes
With Exercise**

What exercise are you getting daily?

_____

_____

_____

How are you monitoring your heart rate?

_____

_____

_____

What are your goals for increasing the amount of
exercise you get regularly?

_____

_____

_____

Where do you see yourself as a more athletic person? Is it on the tennis court? Is it horseback riding? Write about the more athletic person you envision yourself to be.

_____

_____

_____

_____

_____

_____

What truly wonderful things have you noticed about God's creation while taking a walk?

_____

_____

_____

_____

_____

_____

_____

A BIBLE CURE PRAYER
FOR YOU

Lord, help me to change my habits. I need Your strength and determination when mine weakens. Give me the desire and motivation I need to succeed. Amen.

Chapter 4

Battle Diabetes
With Weight Loss

H ave you been battling a weight problem all of
your life with little or no success? No one has
to tell you that many cases of diabetes are directly
linked to obesity. Determine right now that, with
God's help, you will get to your ideal weight and
stay there. Perhaps you've been overweight for so
long that you've given up. In the back of your
mind you may even be thinking, *It's impossible
for me to lose weight.*

The Bible says,
"Nothing is impossible
with God" (Luke 1:37).
It may seem virtually
impossible for you
alone. But you are not

> *Whatever you eat or
> drink or whatever
> you do, you must do
> all for the glory of
> God.*
> —1 CORINTHIANS 10:31

alone! God is on your side, and His strength is available to help you.

Don't even try to face this issue alone. You don't have to. At this moment, whisper a prayer with me asking God to strengthen you to overcome any sense of defeat and bondage that obesity has caused in your life.

A Bible Cure Prayer
FOR YOU

Lord, I surrender the entire issue of weight control to You. Help me to face this issue in my life and find new hope, fresh vision and powerful victory in You. Your Word says, "Nothing is impossible with God." I choose to believe Your Word right now above my feelings of defeat in the arena of weight control. Thank You for loving me just as I am. And thank You for helping me to control my weight so that I will live a longer and better life. Amen.

A Powerful Key to Prevention

Weight control is a powerful key to the prevention of diabetes. Type 2 diabetes is directly linked to obesity and diets rich in saturated fats. Since it is far better to avoid diabetes altogether rather than to contract the disease and ask God to heal you afterward, I strongly encourage you to lose weight if necessary if you are seeking to prevent diabetes. If you already have Type 2 diabetes, weight control is absolutely essential.

Your Ideal Weight—Catch the Vision!

Close your eyes and picture yourself walking around in the body that God intended for you to have—the thin one. You don't have to shop in plus-size stores anymore. You move easily and confidently and no longer huff and puff when you climb stairs. You wear a bathing suit with comfort and confidence. Are you catching the vision?

Following is a chart of your goal weight. Find your height and frame size and write down your goal weight in the space provided.

My goal weight is ____ pounds.
My actual weight is ____ pounds.
I need to lose ___ pounds.

Height and Weight Table for Women

Height	Small Frame	Medium Frame	Large Frame
4'10"	102–111 lbs.	109–121 lbs.	118–131 lbs.
4'11"	103–113 lbs.	111–123 lbs.	120–134 lbs.
5'0"	104–115 lbs.	113–126 lbs.	122–137 lbs.
5'1"	106–118 lbs.	115–129 lbs.	125–140 lbs.
5'2"	108–121 lbs.	118–132 lbs.	128–143 lbs.
5'3"	111–124 lbs.	121–135 lbs.	131–147 lbs.
5'4"	114–127 lbs.	124–138 lbs.	134–151 lbs.
5'5"	117–130 lbs.	127–141 lbs.	137–155 lbs.
5'6"	120–133 lbs.	130–144 lbs.	140–159 lbs.
5'7"	123–136 lbs.	133–147 lbs.	143–163 lbs.
5'8"	126–139 lbs.	136–150 lbs.	146–167 lbs.
5'9"	129–142 lbs.	139–153 lbs.	149–170 lbs.
5'10"	132–145 lbs.	142–156 lbs.	152–173 lbs.
5'11"	135–148 lbs.	145–159 lbs.	155–176 lbs.
6'0"	138–151 lbs.	148–162 lbs.	158–179 lbs.

Height and Weight Table for Men

Height	Small Frame	Medium Frame	Large Frame
5'2"	128–134 lbs.	131–141 lbs.	138–150 lbs.
5'3"	130–136 lbs.	133–143 lbs.	140–153 lbs.
5'4"	132–138 lbs.	135–145 lbs.	142–156 lbs.
5'5"	134–140 lbs.	137–148 lbs.	144–160 lbs.
5'6"	136–142 lbs.	139–151 lbs.	146–164 lbs.
5'7"	138–145 lbs.	142–154 lbs.	149–168 lbs.
5'8"	140–148 lbs.	145–157 lbs.	152–172 lbs.
5'9"	142–151 lbs.	148–160 lbs.	155–176 lbs.
5'10"	144–154 lbs.	151–163 lbs.	158–180 lbs.
5'11"	146–157 lbs.	154–166 lbs.	161–184 lbs.
6'0"	149–160 lbs.	157–170 lbs.	164–188 lbs.
6'1"	152–164 lbs.	160–174 lbs.	168–192 lbs.
6'2"	155–168 lbs.	164–178 lbs.	172–197 lbs.
6'3"	158–172 lbs.	167–182 lbs.	176–202 lbs.
6'4"	162–176 lbs.	171–187 lbs.	181–207 lbs.

Faith Moves Mountains

Feel like you've got a mountain of extra weight to lose? Don't be discouraged. You did not gain it overnight, and losing it overnight would not be healthy. Jesus Christ taught that any mountain of bondage will move when faith is applied. Look at the verse: "I assure you, even if you had faith as small as a mustard seed you could say to this mountain, 'Move from here to there,' and it would move. Nothing would be impossible" (Matt. 17:20).

Let me teach you something about faith. Faith is the most powerful force in the universe. Absolutely nothing is impossible to a person with faith. But listen carefully: Faith is not a feeling or an emotion. It is a choice—a decision to believe God's Word despite everything else to the contrary. I have watched faith move many mountains. I have seen many people rise from wheelchairs and be healed by the power of the Holy Spirit. They were no different than you. They had no less doubt or discouragement. They didn't think higher thoughts or come from more godly families. However, they did choose to believe God. It's so simple.

Choose faith and apply it right now to this bondage.

A BIBLE CURE PRAYER
FOR YOU

Lord Jesus, I choose to believe that the power of the cross is greater than my bondage to obesity. You love me and died on the cross to free me from all of my bondages. I, (your name), choose faith today (date). I give You these (how many pounds) pounds—my mountain of obesity. In Jesus' name I declare victory today! Amen.

Daily Weight Loss Steps

This Bible cure combines faith in God with practical steps, as you know by now. So, here is the practical side: the diet. I recommend you use the rules of good nutrition for diabetics outlined in the previous chapter on nutrition and create a daily diet using these menu planning tips.

Menu Planning Tips

Sample Menu	*Improved Higher Fiber Menu*
BREAKFAST	**BREAKFAST**
$\frac{1}{2}$ cup orange juice	$\frac{1}{2}$ cup orange juice
1 piece whole-grain toast	1 oz. Fiber one
1 tbsp. cream cheese	$\frac{1}{2}$ banana
1 cup skim milk	1 cup skim milk
LUNCH	**LUNCH**
2 oz. chicken salad on	2 oz. chicken salad on
2 slices whole-grain bread	2 slices whole wheat bread
$\frac{1}{2}$ cup carrot sticks	1 small apple
1 glass green tea with Stevia	$\frac{1}{2}$ cup carrot sticks
	1 glass green tea with Stevia
DINNER	**DINNER**
3 oz. grilled salmon	3 oz. grilled salmon
$\frac{1}{2}$ cup broccoli	$\frac{1}{2}$ cup broccoli
1 whole-grain roll	1 serving brown rice
1 tsp. butter or Smart Balance	2 tsp. butter or Smart Balance
$\frac{1}{2}$ cup strawberries	$\frac{1}{2}$ cup strawberries
1 cup head lettuce with	1 cup Romaine lettuce with
2 tbsp. French dressing	2 tbsp. French dressing
1 cup skim milk	1 cup skim milk
SNACKS	**SNACKS**
6 oz. yogurt	2 cups melon
1 apple	1 apple

Simple Rules

The following are simple dieting rules that I always recommend to my patients who need to lose weight.

1. Graze throughout the day. (Eat lots of salads and veggies often throughout the day.)
2. Eat a fairly large breakfast.
3. Eat smaller mid-morning, mid-afternoon and evening snacks.
4. Avoid all simple sugar foods such as candies, cookies, cakes, pies and doughnuts. If you must have sugar, use either Stevia or Sweet Balance (found in health food stores.)
5. Drink two quarts of filtered or bottled water a day. It is best to drink two 8-oz. glasses 30 minutes before each meal, or one to two 8-oz. glasses 2½ hours after each meal.
6. Avoid alcohol.
7. Avoid all fried foods.
8. Avoid, or decrease dramatically, starches. Starches include all breads,

crackers, bagels, potatoes, pasta, rice, corn, black beans, pinto beans and red beans. Also limit your intake of bananas.

9. Eat fresh fruits; steamed, stir-fried or raw vegetables; lean meats; salads preferably with extra-virgin olive oil and vinegar; nuts (almonds, organic peanuts) and seeds.

10. Take fiber supplements such as Fiber Plus, Perdiem Fiber or any other fiber without NutraSweet or sugar.

11. Take 2 tablespoons of milk of magnesia each day if constipated. However, first make sure you are consuming at least 35 grams of fiber each day and drinking 2–3 quarts of water a day.

12. For snacks, choose Iron Man PR Bars, Zone Bars or Balance Bars. My favorite snack bar is the yogurt honey peanut Balance Bars. These may be purchased at a health food store.

13. Do not eat past 7 P.M.

Start every day with prayer to God for success. Speak aloud the Bible verses that are scattered throughout this booklet. In addition, plan your menu

> *For God has not given us a spirit of fear and timidity, but of power, love, and self-discipline.*
> —2 TIMOTHY 1:7

each day and follow these additional simple rules. With a little patience, you'll be well on your way to that slimmer person you pictured when you closed your eyes—the healthy person God intended you to be!

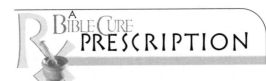

R **A BIBLE CURE PRESCRIPTION**

Create a Sample Menu

Step 1: Start with prayer for success.

Step 2: Select a victory verse.

Step 3: Today's menu based upon the menu planning tips:

Breakfast: _____

_____

_____

Lunch: _____

_____

_____

Dinner: _____

_____

_____

Snacks: _____

_____

_____

In addition, I will implement the following simple rules:

❑ Graze throughout the day. (Eat lots of salads and veggies often throughout the day.)

❑ Eat a fairly large breakfast.

❑ Eat smaller mid-morning, mid-afternoon and evening snacks.

❑ Avoid all simple sugar foods such as candies, cookies, cakes, pies and doughnuts.

❑ Drink two quarts of filtered or bottled water a day.

❑ Other: _____

_____

_____

_____

_____

_____

Chapter 5

Battle Diabetes With Nutrients and Supplements

As you battle diabetes, you will discover that nutrients are also very helpful in controlling your blood sugar. There are God-created ways for you to add nutrients and supplements to your diet to begin controlling your blood sugar in a systematic, natural way. Following is a list of nutrients and supplements that will help you fight diabetes.

Chromium. I recommend that you take chromium. Why? Research suggests that our bodies require certain nutrients for normal blood sugar and insulin absorption. Chromium is one of those nutrients. Thirteen out of fifteen studies demonstrated that chromium supplementation worked effectively in maintaining blood sugar levels with a minimum of insulin.[1]

Chromium in the form of chromium polynicotinate in a dose of at least 200 micrograms (mcgs) a day helps improve glucose tolerance in both Type 1 and Type 2 diabetics. Chromium also helps to improve the processing of glucose in patients whose glucose intolerance is a pre-diabetic syndrome, as well as the processing of glucose in women who have gestational diabetes.[2]

Mild chromium deficiency is quite common in the U.S. because the amounts of chromium in our diets can be depleted by excessive amounts of processed foods, especially white sugar and flour.

> *Do not carouse with drunkards and gluttons, for they are on their way to poverty. Too much sleep clothes a person with rags.*
> —Proverbs 23:20–21

Chromium actually helps to increase the efficiency of insulin; it allows insulin to more effectively transport the glucose into the cells.

I do not recommend, however, that patients take chromium picolinate since it has been linked to chromosomal damage in rats. I do recommend instead chromium polynicotinate. The dose is usually 200 micrograms, two to three times a day.

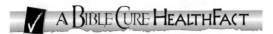

Chrome-Plated Protection

The trace mineral chromium has been shown to improve the body's ability to regulate blood sugar, says Richard A. Anderson, Ph.D., with the U.S. Department of Agriculture's Human Nutrition Research Center in Maryland. He lists the following foods as containing trace chromium:

- Broccoli
- Grapefruit
- Fortified breakfast cereals
- Turkey

You can boost your chromium supplies by eating these foods. One cup of broccoli contains 22 micrograms, which is 18 percent of the DV. ("DV" refers to Daily Values, a shorthand version of the Food and Nutrition Board's Recommended Dietary Allowances that you see on food labels.) A 2.5-oz. waffle has almost 7 micrograms, which is 6 percent of the DV; and a 3-oz. serving of turkey ham has 10 micrograms, or 8 percent of the DV.[3]

HEALTHFACT HEALTHFACT HEALTHFACT HEALTHFACT HEALTHFACT HEALTHFACT HEALTHFACT

Alpha-lipoic acid is a very powerful antioxidant. It has been used for many years in Europe to improve diabetic neuropathy, usually at an intake of 300 milligrams, two to three times a day. Lipoic acid may also help to lower blood sugar, especially when in combination with chromium. I recommend taking 300 milligrams of lipoic acid two to three times a day.

However, if you are taking diabetic medications, you should monitor your blood sugar closely since lipoic acid and chromium are able to lower blood sugar quite significantly. You should also be followed closely by your medical doctor.

Vitamin E. Antioxidants are extremely important in all diabetic patients. Vitamin E in high doses (usually at least 800 International Units) may improve glucose tolerance with Type 2 diabetes. In other words, it improves the action of insulin and thus helps to lower the blood sugar. Vitamin E will help protect diabetics from developing cataracts, as well as protect their blood vessels from the damaging effects of diabetes.

Vitamin C. Most patients with diabetes also have low vitamin C levels. Diabetics tend to have elevated sorbitol levels. Sorbitol is a form of sugar that can accumulate in the body and thus damage the nerves, eyes and kidneys. Vitamin C is able to effectively lower the level of sorbitol, thus preventing these long-term complications.

You should take at least 2,000 milligrams of vitamin C a day. I personally prefer the effervescent vitamin C known as Emergen-C. Most diabetics do not have enough vitamin C inside the blood cells since insulin is needed to help transport the vitamin C into the cells. This low level of vitamin C inside the blood cell can lead to vascular disease and tendencies toward bleeding. I recommend taking 1 gram of effervescent vitamin C at least two to three times per day.

Magnesium. Magnesium levels also tend to be low in diabetics. Adequate magnesium intake may improve insulin production in elderly patients. It may also prevent long-term complications of diabetes such as heart disease and diabetic retinopathy. Diabetics usually need at least 700–800 milligrams of magnesium per day, whereas the Recommended Daily Allowance (RDA) for magnesium in an adult male is only 350 milligrams a day.

The best dietary sources of magnesium include the following:

- Seeds and nuts
- Whole grains
- Legumes
- Baked halibut
- Steamed oysters (some health experts recommend avoiding oysters altogether)
- Dark green leafy vegetables
- Long-grain brown rice

If you decide to use a magnesium supplement, choose either magnesium aspartate, magnesium glycinate, magnesium taurate or magnesium citrate. Taking too much magnesium can cause diarrhea, however, so start with only 400 milligrams of magnesium a day and increase the dosage slowly.

Zinc. Diabetics commonly have low levels of zinc. Type 2 diabetics tend to lose zinc in their urine. Zinc is very important in the synthesis of insulin. Zinc, as well as magnesium, is also found in nuts, seeds, legumes and whole grains. However, one should take at least 30 milligrams of zinc a day. This should be balanced with at least 2–3 milligrams of copper a day.

A comprehensive multivitamin like Theragram-M will contain adequate doses of these vitamins and minerals, including magnesium, zinc and copper.

Niacin. Niacin in the form of niacinamide may be beneficial in Type 1 diabetes if the disease is detected early enough. This B vitamin may help to restore the insulin-producing cells in the pancreas, which are the beta cells. A good dose is approximately 500 milligrams in adults with Type 1 diabetes. However, you must have your liver functions checked by a physician at least once every three months while on niacin.

Patients with Type 2 diabetes (which is non-insulin dependent) may benefit from smaller amounts of niacin, such as 250–500 milligrams a day. High doses of niacin, such as 2–3 grams a day, may actually raise the blood sugar in patients with Type 2 diabetes.

Vitamin B$_6$. Vitamin B$_6$ may prevent diabetic neuropathy. If you recall from an earlier discussion, diabetic neuropathy causes tingling sensations, numbness, pain, muscle weakness and eventual loss of function of extremities due to long-term diabetes affecting the peripheral nerves. A dose of 50–100 milligrams of vitamin B$_6$ a day may aid in preventing diabetic neuropathy. Also, vitamin B$_6$ aids magnesium in getting inside the cell where it can help prevent heart disease and diabetic retinopathy in diabetic patients. B$_{12}$ may also be beneficial in treating diabetic neuropathy when taken in a dose of 1,000 micrograms per day.

Biotin. Biotin is another B vitamin that is needed to process glucose. Sixteen milligrams of biotin a day may decrease blood sugar levels dramatically. However, you should be monitoring your blood sugars throughout the day in order to prevent hypoglycemia, which is low blood sugar.

Essential fatty acids are also very important

for diabetics. *Gamma-linolenic acid* (GLA) is found in black currant oil, evening primrose oil and borage oil. GLA may protect a diabetic from developing diabetic neuropathy. You should take approximately 240 milligrams of GLA per day.

Omega-3 fatty acids are found in flaxseed oil and fatty fish such as salmon, mackerel, herring and halibut. Omega-3 fatty acids help prevent arteriosclerosis and aid in insulin secretion in Type 2 diabetics.

However, fish oil supplements may actually worsen diabetes in Type 2 diabetics and should be avoided. (Use flaxseed oil instead.) Eat at least two to three 3.5-ounce servings of fatty fish per week and/or take 1 tablespoon or 7 capsules of flaxseed oil per day. Flaxseed oil should be refrigerated once it is opened.

Gymnema sylvestre is an herb from India that is effective in both Type 1 and Type 2 diabetes. Gymnema helps the pancreas produce insulin in Type 2 diabetes and helps lower the blood sugar in both Type 1 and Type 2 diabetes by enhancing the action of insulin. The recommended dose of gymnema is 400 milligrams a day.

Billberry is a plant found in Europe that helps improve the circulation to the retina, thus helping to prevent diabetic retinopathy (the most common cause of blindness in the U.S.). I believe all diabetics should be taking billberry on a daily basis. The normal dose is 80 milligrams, three times a day. Billberry may also decrease the risk of developing diabetic cataracts.

Quercetin is a bioflavonoid that may also reduce the risk of both diabetic retinopathy and cataracts. Approximately 1 gram of quercetin per day would prove very beneficial.

Grapeseed extract is another bioflavonoid similar to quercetin that can strengthen the small blood vessels of the retina and thus prevent diabetic retinopathy. I recommend 50 milligrams of grapeseed or pine bark extract two to four times a day.

Ginkgo biloba improves blood flow to the brain as well as to the arms, fingers, legs and toes. Peripheral vascular disease (where the blood supply to the lower extremities is less than

> *Praise the LORD, I tell myself; with my whole heart, I will praise his holy name. Praise the LORD, I tell myself, and never forget the good things he does for me. He forgives all my sins and heals all my diseases.*
> —PSALM 103:1–3

normal) is very common in long-term diabetics, so improving blood flow is critical in these patients. I recommend 100 milligrams of ginkgo biloba, three times a day in order to improve blood flow.

Bitter melon is a fruit found in South America, Africa and Asia and is very effective in lowering blood sugar when taken in the freshly juiced form. The juice, however, is extremely bitter; very few patients are able to take it consistently. High doses of bitter melon juice can also cause diarrhea and abdominal pain. Usually 2 ounces of bitter melon juice per day is sufficient.

> *Words satisfy the soul as food satisfies the stomach; the right words on a person's lips bring satisfaction. Those who love to talk will experience the consequences, for the tongue can kill or nourish life.*
> —PROVERBS 18:20–21

As you have observed, there are many nutrients and supplements that can help you effectively battle diabetes. Regularly consult with your physician and use these vitamins and nutrients as he or she may recommend. God has created these wonderful natural substances to empower us in maintaining good health and overcoming the debilitating effects of diabetes.

Try a Comprehensive Supplement

If you're like many people, trying to keep track of all of these vitamins and minerals can seem overwhelming. Do not be concerned. Many of the vitamins and minerals listed above can be taken in a comprehensive multivitamin and mineral supplement. You can find a good supplement in any health food store. I encourage you to include an antioxidant supplement as well. Check the label to be sure it has the following:

- At least 400 mg. of magnesium

- 1,000 mcg. of B_{12}

- 100 mg. of B_6

- 20 to 30 mg. of zinc

- 800 I.U. of natural vitamin E

- 1,000 mg. of vitamin C (I also recommend

the powdered effervescent form such as Emergen-C).

A Final Note

As my patients with Type 2 diabetes follow this program and monitor their blood sugar, they find that their blood sugar usually comes down to within normal range in a few months. Until they receive complete divine healing from God, my Type 1 diabetics will always be on insulin. However, many times they are able to lower their dosage of insulin by following the measures outlined in this booklet.

Battling Diabetes With
Nutrients and Supplements

Check which of the following nutrients or supplements you are presently taking. Circle the ones you will consult with your physician about taking.

❑ Chromium polynicolinate (200 mcg., 2–3 times a day)

❑ Alpha-lipoic acid (300 mg., 2–3 times a day)

❑ Vitamin E (800 I.U. daily mixed tocopherols or natural varieties, avoid synthetic forms)

❑ Vitamin C (2,000 mg. daily)

❑ Magnesium (400–800 mg. daily)

❑ Zinc (30 mg. daily, balanced with at least 2–3 mgs of copper daily)

- ❏ Vitamin B_6 (50–100 mg. daily)

- ❏ Vitamin B_{12} (1,000 mcg. daily)

- ❏ Biotin (8–16 mg. daily while monitoring blood sugars closely)

- ❏ GLA (240 mg. daily)

- ❏ Gymnema sylvestre (400 mg. daily)

- ❏ Billberry (80 mg., 3 times a day)

- ❏ Quercetin (1 g. daily)

- ❏ Grapeseed or pine bark extract (50 mg., 2–4 times a day)

- ❏ Gingko biloba (100 mg., 3 times a day)

- ❏ Bitter melon (2 oz. daily)

- ❏ Niacin (250–500 mg. daily with a check-up at least once every three months of liver function)

A BIBLE CURE PRAYER
FOR YOU

Heavenly Father, help me apply these things I have learned in my battle against diabetes. Help me eat wisely and obtain my ideal body weight. Show me which vitamins, minerals and supplements will best help my body fight diabetes. Heal my body so that insulin will be produced and then used by my cells in a healthy way. Strengthen my resolve to exercise regularly. Thank You for making me so wonderfully. Keep me in Your divine health so that I may live a long, productive life serving You. Amen.

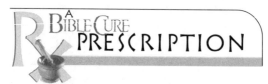

Winning the Battle Over Diabetes

What starches have you reduced or eliminated from your diet?

_____

What fruits do you eat?

_____

_____

What natural sweeteners do you use?

_____

List the vitamins, minerals and supplements you now take.

_____

_____

Describe your regular form of exercise.

_____

_____

A PERSONAL NOTE

From Don and Mary Colbert

God desires to heal you of disease. His Word is full of promises that confirm His love for you and His desire to give you His abundant life. His desire includes more than physical health for you; He wants to make you whole in your mind and spirit as well through a personal relationship with His Son, Jesus Christ.

If you haven't met my best friend, Jesus, I would like to take this opportunity to introduce Him to you. It is very simple.

If you are ready to let Him come into your heart and become your best friend, just bow your head and sincerely pray this prayer from your heart:

Lord Jesus, I want to know You as my Savior and Lord. I believe You are the Son of God and that You died for my sins. I also believe You were raised from the dead and now sit at the right hand of the Father praying for me. I ask You to forgive me for my sins and change my heart so that I can

*be Your child and live with You eternally.
Thank You for Your peace. Help me to
walk with You so that I can begin to know
You as my best friend and my Lord. Amen.*

If you have prayed this prayer, we rejoice
with you in your decision and your new relationship with Jesus. Please contact us at
pray4me@strang.com so that we can send you
some materials that will help you become estab-
lished in your relationship with the Lord. You
have just made the most important decision of
your life. We look forward to hearing from you.

Appendix A

The Balanced
Carb-Protein-Fat Plan

There is no perfect diet for everyone. A regimen that's healthy for one individual may actually be harmful to another due to food allergies, food sensitivities, gastrointestinal disturbances, blood types and other factors.

The diet of the majority of people in the United States contains excessive amounts of fat, sugar, salt and starch, and it has a significant lack of fiber. The keys to the ultimate healthy lifestyle are found in eating primarily fruits, vegetables, whole grains, nuts, seeds, beans, legumes and lean meats.

Avoid refined sugar and flour; avoid fats, which include hydrogenated fats, saturated fats and heat processed polyunsaturated fats such as luncheon meats, cured meats and sausage; and avoid foods high in salt. Also, limit your intake of red meat, choosing the leanest cuts possible.

The nutritional plan I recommend to my patients is the Balanced Carb-Protein-Fat Plan. Here's how it works. Each time you eat you should combine foods in a ratio of 40 percent carbohydrates, 30 percent proteins and 30 percent fats.

This program balances the correct ratio of carbohydrates, proteins and fats, thereby controlling insulin.

Elevated insulin levels decrease physical performance and are one of the primary predictors used in evaluating a person's risk of developing heart disease. To simplify this program, I will list the food categories and blocks, and then demonstrate how to use the blocks through the day. Let's look at some comparisons.

- One block of protein is equal to 7 grams of protein, which is equivalent to approximately 1 oz. of meat, such as beef, chicken breast, turkey breast and so on.

- One block of carbohydrates is equal to 9 grams of carbohydrates, which is equivalent to ½ slice of bread, ¼ bagel, ⅕ cup of rice, ⅓ banana, ½ apple or ¼ cup of pasta.

This will be explained in greater detail later.

- One block of fat is equal to 1½ grams of fat, which is equivalent to ⅓ tsp. of olive oil, 6 peanuts, 3 almonds, 1 tbsp. of avocado and so on.

You will be getting much larger portion sizes than each individual food block. In fact, the average sedentary woman will get three food blocks at each meal plus one food block midmorning, one food block midafternoon and one food block at bedtime. An active female who exercises three to four times a week for at least thirty minutes, may have four food blocks with each meal and one food block between meals and at bedtime.

A sedentary male may have four food blocks at each meal and one food block between meals and at bedtime, whereas the active male, who exercises three to four times a week, may have five to six food blocks at each meal and one food block between meals and at bedtime.

Let's discuss the different food blocks—starting with protein.

Protein Blocks

(Approximately 7 grams of protein for each block)

Meats

One ounce of skinless chicken breast, skinless turkey breast or free range chicken. Or 1 ounce of skinless dark meat of turkey, skinless dark meat of chicken, hamburger with less than 10 percent fat, lean pork chop, lean ham, lean Canadian bacon, lean lamb or veal. Note: I do not recommend eating pork and ham regularly. If an individual has a degenerative disease, he or she should avoid these meats completely.

Fish

Eat 1½ oz. of the following:

Salmon	Mackerel
Orange roughy	Red snapper
Sole	Mahi-mahi
Trout	Halibut
Grouper	

Eggs, dairy products and soy protein

Eggs—one whole egg or three egg whites
Dairy products—1 oz. low-fat cheese, ¼ cup of low-fat cottage cheese
Soy protein—⅓ oz. of protein powder, ¼ soy burger, 3 oz. of tofu

Carbohydrate Blocks

(Approximately 9 grams of carbohydrates for each block)

Fruit

1 tangerine, lemon, lime, kiwi or peach
½ apple, orange, grapefruit, pear or nectarine
⅓ banana
1 cup strawberries, raspberries
⅓ cup cubed watermelon, cubed cantaloupe
½ cup cubed honeydew melon, cherries, black-
berries, blueberries, grapes, cubed pineapples,
papaya
⅓ cup applesauce, mango

Juice

¼ cup grape, pineapple
⅓ cup apple, grapefruit, orange, lemon
¾ cup V8

Cooked Vegetables

⅛ cup baked beans
⅕ cup sweet potatoes or mashed potatoes
¼ cup lentils, kidney beans, black beans, red
beans, lima beans, pinto beans, refried beans,
corn
⅓ cup peas, baked potato
1 cup asparagus, green beans, carrots
1¼ cup broccoli, spinach, squash
1⅓ cup cabbage

Cooked Vegetables
1½ cup zucchini, Brussels sprouts, eggplant
1¾ cup turnip greens
2 cups cauliflower, collard greens

Raw Vegetables
1 cucumber
2 tomatoes
1 cup onions (chopped), snow peas
1½ cup broccoli
2 cups cauliflower
2½ cups celery, green peppers (chopped)
3 cups cabbage, mushrooms (chopped)
4 cups romaine lettuce (chopped), cucumber
(sliced)
6 cups spinach

Grains
⅓ oz. brown or white rice
⅓ cup cooked pasta
⅓ cup cooked oatmeal (or ½ oz. dry), or grits
¼ bagel, English muffin
½ biscuit, waffle, or ½ of a 4-inch pancake,
flour tortilla
½ oz. dry cereal
1 rice cake or corn tortilla
4 saltine crackers

High-Sugar Items
½ tbsp. honey or molasses
2 tsp. maple syrup
2 tbsp. ketchup, jelly (choose fructose jelly)

Fat Blocks

⅓ tsp. almond butter, olive oil, canola oil, flaxseed oil
⅓ tsp. natural peanut butter
1 tsp. olive oil and vinegar dressing, light may-
onnaise, chopped walnuts
1 tbsp. avocado, guacamole
1 whole macadamia nut
1½ tsp. almond (slivered)
3 almonds, olives, pistachios, cashews
6 peanuts

The Basics

An example of a meal with four food blocks would
be 4 oz. of chicken (equal to four protein blocks);
1 cup of cooked asparagus, 1 head of lettuce and
1 cup of red beans (all together equal to four carbohydrates blocks); 1 tablespoon of olive oil and
vinegar dressing (equal to four fat blocks).

To simplify this meal plan even more, picture
the palm of your hand and imagine placing a
piece of protein (such as a piece of chicken,
turkey, fish or lean red meat) the size of your

palm. Next cup your hands and picture putting in the amount of vegetables or fruit that you can hold. You should add 12 almonds, 12 cashews or 12 pistachio nuts or 24 peanuts. You are holding the ingredients for your healthy meal.

It's best to dramatically limit starches, which include bread, bagels, crackers, pasta, rice, pretzels, popcorn, beans, cereals, corn, potatoes, potato chips, corn chips and any other starchy item. I recommend grazing through the day, eating a fairly large breakfast, lunch and dinner and smaller midmorning, midafternoon and evening snacks. Eat the evening meal before 7 P.M.

People who have degenerative diseases such as heart disease, high blood pressure, high cholesterol, diabetes, hypoglycemia, cancer or patients who desire optimal health should closely follow the Balanced Carb-Protein-Fat Plan program.

If the Balanced Carb-Protein-Fat Plan program seems too complicated for you, simply follow these basic instructions:

1. Reduce the intake of high starch foods, including bread, crackers, bagels, pretzels, corn, popcorn, potatoes,

sweet potatoes, potato chips, pasta, rice, beans and bananas. Better yet, eliminate them all together.

2. Avoid all simple sugar food such as candies, cookies, cakes, pies and donuts. If you must have sugar use Sweet Balance or Stevia, a sweetener made from kiwi fruit. Choose fruit instead of fruit juices.

3. Increase your intake of nonstarchy vegetables such as spinach, lettuce, cabbage, broccoli, asparagus, green beans and cauliflower.

4. Choose healthy proteins such as turkey breast, chicken breast, fish, free-range beef, low-fat cottage cheese and so on. Select healthy fats such as nuts, seeds, flaxseed oil, extra-virgin olive oil or small amounts of organic butter. Use extra-virgin olive oil and vinegar as a salad dressing. Choose the healthy fats we have listed instead of polyunsaturated, saturated and hydrogenated fats.

5. Eat three meals a day consisting of fruit, nonstarchy vegetables, lean meat and good fat. You should also have a healthy midmorning, midafternoon and evening snack.

By following these guidelines I believe you will experience increased energy and improved health.

Notes

PREFACE
THERE'S HOPE FOR DIABETES

1. M. Sommers, S. Johnson, et al. *Davis's Manual of Nursing Therapeutics for Diseases and Disorders* (n.p., F. A. Davis Co., 1997), 332.

CHAPTER 1
KNOW YOUR ENEMY

1. Sommers, *Davis's Manual of Nursing Therapeutics for Diseases and Disorders,* 332.
2. National Diabetes Data Group, National Institutes of Health, *Diabetes in America,* 2nd Edition. (Bethesda, MD: National Institutes of Health, 1995).

CHAPTER 2
BATTLE DIABETES WITH GOOD NUTRITION

1. Statistics obtained in 1999 from the Web site www.4BetterHealth.com

CHAPTER 5
BATTLE DIABETES WITH NUTRIENTS AND SUPPLEMENTS

1. Walter Mertz, "Chromium in Human Nutrition: A Review," *Journal of Nutrition 123* (1993): 626–633.
2. G. W. Evans, "The Effect of Chromium Picolinate on Insulin Control Parameters in Humans" *International Journal of Biosocial Medical Research II* (1989): 163–180.
3. Adapted from Selene Yeager, *New Foods for Healing* (Emmaus, PA: Rodale Press, Inc. 1998), 186.

Don Colbert, M.D., was born in Tupelo, Mississippi. He attended Oral Roberts School of Medicine in Tulsa, Oklahoma, where he received a bachelor of science degree in biology in addition to his degree in medicine. Dr. Colbert completed his internship and residency with Florida Hospital in Orlando, Florida. He is board certified in family practice and has received extensive training in nutritional medicine.

If you would like more
information about natural and
divine healing, or information about
Divine Health Nutritional Products®,
you may contact
Dr. Colbert at:

DR. DON COLBERT

1908 Boothe Circle
Longwood, FL 32750
Telephone: 407-331-7007
(For ordering products only)

Dr. Colbert's website is
www.drcolbert.com.

Disclaimer: Dr. Colbert and the staff of Divine Health Wellness Center are prohibited from addressing a patient's medical condition by phone, facsimile or e-mail. Please refer questions related to your medical condition to your own primary care physician.

Announcing

Divine Health Diabetic Support

Proper nutrition is the cornerstone to managing your diabetes. Put your trust in the Lord, for He will help you to overcome any obstacle. Exercise and weight control hold special benefits for diabetics. God wants you to look and feel you're very best!

Diabetes is the seventh leading cause of death among Americans. Tragically, most individuals diagnosed with Type II diabetes may have been able to prevent the onset of the disease with proper nutrition and exercise. Divine Health Diabetic Support was formulated to help your body improve insulin sensitivity and maintain an optimal fasting glucose level. Our Diabetic Support formula contains 300 mg lipoic acid, 400 mg of gymnema leaf extract, 800 mcg of chromium and 3000 mcg of biotin. These herbs and botanicals are used for their hypoglycemic and insulin modifying effects.

Recommended dosage: Oone capsule two to three times a day

* Divine Health Lipoic Acid can be used for added support.
Product # 035 – 60 Capsules